# Table of Contents

# INTRODUCTION

Nutrition is the study of nutrients in food, how the body uses them, and the relationship between diet, health, and disease. Nutritionists use ideas from molecular biology, biochemistry, and genetics to understand how nutrients affect the human body. Nutrition also focuses on how people can use dietary choices to reduce the risk of disease, what happens if a person has too much or too little of a nutrient, and how allergies work. Nutrients provide nourishment. Proteins, carbohydrates, fat, vitamins, minerals, fiber, and water are all nutrients. If people do not have the right balance of nutrients in their diet, their risk of developing certain health conditions increases.

# MACRONUTRIENTS

Consuming the right balance of nutrients can help maintain a healthful lifestyle.

Macronutrients are nutrients that people need in relatively large quantities.

## Carbohydrates

Sugar, starch, and fiber are types of carbohydrates.

Sugars are simple carbs. The body quickly breaks down and absorbs sugars and processed starch. They can provide rapid energy, but they do not leave a person feeling full. They can also cause a spike in blood sugar levels. Frequent sugar spikes increase the risk of type 2 diabetes and its complications.

Fiber is also a carbohydrate. The body breaks down some types of fiber and uses them for energ; others are metabolized by gut bacteria, while other types pass through the body. Fiber and unprocessed starch are complex carbs. It takes the body some time to break down and absorb complex carbs. After eating fiber, a person will feel full for longer. Fiber may also reduce the risk of diabetes, cardiovascular disease, and colorectal cancer. Complex carbs are a more healthful choice than sugars and refined carbs.

## Proteins

Proteins consist of amino acids, which are organic compounds that occur naturally. There are 20 amino acids. Some of these are essentialTrusted Source, which means people need to obtain them from food. The body can make the others. Some foods provide complete protein, which means they contain all the essential amino acids the body needs. Other foods contain various combinations of amino acids. Most plant-based foods do not contain complete protein, so a person who follows a vegan diet needs to eat a range of foods throughout the day that provides the essential amino acids.

## Fats

Fats are essential for:

- lubricating joints

- helping organs produce hormones

- enabling the body to absorb certain vitamins

- reducing inflammation

- preserving brain health

Too much fat can lead to obesity, high cholesterol, liver disease, and other health problems.

However, the type of fat a person eats makes a difference. Unsaturated fats, such as olive oil, are more healthful than saturated fats, which tend to come from animals.

## Water

The adult human body is up to 60% water, and it needs water for many processes. Water contains no calories, and it does not provide energy. Many people recommend consuming 2 liters, or 8 glasses, of water a day, but it can also come from dietary sources, such as fruit and vegetables. Adequate hydration will result in pale yellow urine. Requirements will also depend on an individual's body size and age, environmental factors, activity levels, health status, and so on.

# MICRONUTRIENTS

Micronutrients are essential in small amounts. They include vitamins and minerals. Manufacturers sometimes add these to foods. Examples include fortified cereals and rice.

Minerals

The body needs carbon, hydrogen, oxygen, and nitrogen. It also needs dietary minerals, such as iron, potassium, and so on. In most cases, a varied and balanced diet will provide the minerals a person needs. If a deficiency occurs, a doctor may recommend supplements. Here are some of the minerals the body needs to function well.

Potassium

Potassium is an electrolyte. It enables the kidneys, the heart, the muscles, and the nerves to work properly. The 2015–2020 Dietary Guidelines for Americans recommend that adults consume 4,700 milligramsTrusted Source (mg) of potassium each day. Too little can lead to high blood pressure, stroke, and kidney stones. Too much may be harmful to people with kidney disease. Avocados, coconut water, bananas, dried fruit, squash, beans, and lentils are good sources.

Sodium

Sodium is an electrolyte that helps:

maintain nerve and muscle function

regulate fluid levels in the body

Too little can lead to hyponatremia. Symptoms include lethargy, confusion, and fatigue. Learn more here. Too much can lead to high blood pressure, which increases the risk of cardiovascular disease and stroke. Table salt, which is made up of sodium and chloride, is a popular condiment. However, most people consume too much sodium, as it already occurs naturally in most foods. Experts urge people not to add table salt to their diet. Current guidelines recommend consuming no more than 2,300 mg of sodium a day, or around one teaspoon. This recommendation includes both naturally-occurring sources, as well as salt a person adds to their food. People with high blood pressure or kidney disease should eat less.

Calcium

The body needs calciumTrusted Source to form bones and teeth. It also supports the nervous system, cardiovascular health, and other functions. Too little can cause bones and teeth to weaken. Symptoms of a severe deficiency include tingling in the fingers and changes in heart rhythm, which can be life-threatening. Too much can lead to constipation, kidney stones, and reduced absorption of other minerals. Current guidelines for adults recommend consuming 1,000 mg a day, and 1,200 mg for women aged 51 and over. Good sources include dairy products, tofu, legumes,and green, leafy vegetables.

Phosphorus

Phosphorus is present in all body cells and contributes toTrusted Source the health of the bones and teeth. Too little phosphorus can lead to bone diseases, affect appetite, muscle strength, and coordination. It can also result in anemia, a higher risk of infection, burning or prickling sensations in the skin, and confusion. Too much in the diet is unlikely to cause health problems though toxicity is possible from supplements, medications, and phosphorus metabolism problems. Adults should aim to consume around 700 mgTrusted Source of phosphorus each day. Good sources include dairy products, salmon, lentils, and cashews.

Magnesium

Magnesium contributes toTrusted Source muscle and nerve function. It helps regulate blood pressure and blood sugar levels, and it enables the body to produce proteins, bone, and DNA. Too little magnesium can eventually lead to weakness, nausea, tiredness, restless legs, sleep conditions, and other symptoms. Too much can result in digestive and, eventually, heart problems. Nuts, spinach, and beans are good sources of magnesium. Adult females need 320 mgTrusted Source of magnesium each day, and adult males need 420 mg.

Zinc

Zinc plays a role in the health of body cells, the immune system, wound healing, and the creation of proteins. Too little can lead to hair loss, skin sores, changes in taste or smell,and diarrhea, but this is rare. Too much can lead to digestive problems and headaches. Click here to learn more. Adult females need 8 mg of zinc a day, and adult males need 11 mg. Dietary sources include oysters, beef, fortified breakfast cereals, and baked beans. For more on dietary sources of zinc, click here.

Iron

Iron is crucial for the formationTrusted Source of red blood cells, which carry oxygen to all parts of the body. It also plays a role in forming connective tissue and creating hormones. Too little can result in anemia, including digestive issues, weakness, and difficulty thinking. Learn more here about iron deficiency. Too much can lead to digestive problems, and very high levels can be fatal.nGood sources include fortified cereals, beef liver, lentils, spinach, and tofu. Adults need 8 mgTrusted Source of iron a day, but females need 18 mg during their reproductive years.

Manganese

The body uses manganese to produce energyTrusted Source, it plays a role in blood clotting, and it supports the immune system. Too little can result in weak bones in children, skin rashes in men, and mood changes in women. Too much can lead to tremors, muscle spasms, and other symptoms, but only with very high amounts. Mussels, hazelnuts, brown rice, chickpeas, and spinach all provide manganese. Male adults need 2.3 mgTrusted Source of manganese each day, and females need 1.8 mg.

Copper

Copper helps the body make energy and produce connective tissues and blood vessels. Too little copper can lead to tiredness, patches of light skin, high cholesterol, and connective tissue disorders. This is rare. Too much copper can result in liver damage, abdominal pain, nausea, and diarrhea. Too much copper also reduces the absorption of zinc. Good sources include beef liver, oysters, potatoes, mushrooms, sesame seeds, and sunflower seeds. Adults need 900 micrograms (mcg) of copper each day.

Selenium

Selenium is made up of over 24 selenoproteins, and it plays a crucial roleTrusted Source in reproductive and thyroid health. As an antioxidant, it can also prevent cell damage. Too much selenium can cause garlic breath, diarrhea, irritability, skin rashes, brittle hair or nails, and other symptoms. Too little can result in heart disease, infertility in men, and arthritis. Adults need 55 mcg of selenium a day. Brazil nuts are an excellent source of selenium. Other plant sources include spinach, oatmeal, and baked beans. Tuna, ham, and enriched macaroni are all excellent sources.

Vitamins

Eating a variety of healthful foods can provide the body with different vitamins.

People need small amounts of various vitamins. Some of these, such as vitamin C, are also antioxidants. This means they help protect cells from damage by removing toxic molecules, known as free radicals, from the body.bVitamins can be:

Water-soluble: The eight B vitamins and vitamin C

Fat-soluble: Vitamins A, D, E, and K

Learn more about vitamins here.

Water soluble vitamins

People need to consume water-soluble vitamins regularly because the body removes them more quickly, and it cannot store them easily.

Vitamin         Effect of too little      Effect of too much      Sources

B-1 Beriberi

Wernicke-Korsakoff syndrome

Unclear, as the body excretes it in the urine.  Fortified cereals and rice, pork, trout, black beans

B-2 (riboflavin) Hormonal problems, skin disorders, swelling in the mouth and throat      Unclear, as the body excretes it in the urine.      Beef liver, breakfast cereal, oats, yogurt, mushrooms, almonds

B-3 (niacin) Pellagra, including skin changes, red tongue, digestive and neurological symptoms Facial flushing, burning, itching, headaches, rashes, and dizziness    Beef liver, chicken breast, brown rice, fortified cereals, peanuts.

B-5 (pantothenic acid) Numbness and burning in hands and feet, fatigue, stomach pain    Digestive problems at high doses. Breakfast cereal, beef liver, shiitake mushroom, sunflower seeds

B-6 (pyridoxamine, pyridoxal) Anemia, itchy rash, skin changes, swollen tongue       Nerve damage, loss of muscle control. Chickpeas, beef liver, tuna, chicken breast, fortified cereals, potatoes

B-7 (biotin) Hair loss, rashes around the eyes and other body openings, conjunctivitis Unclear.   Beef liver, egg, salmon, sunflower seeds, sweet potato

B-9 (folic acid, folateTrusted Source)        Weakness, fatigue, difficulty focusing, heart palpitations, shortness of breath  May increase cancer risk      Beef liver, spinach, black-eyed peas, fortified cereal, asparagus

B-12 (cobalamins). Anemia, fatigue, constipation, weight loss, neurological changes    No adverse effects reported       Clams, beef liver, fortified yeasts, plant milks, and breakfast cereals, some oily fish.

Vitamin C (ascorbic acid( . Scurvy, including fatigue, skin rash, gum inflammation, poor wound healing       Nausea, diarrhea, stomach cramps      Citrus fruits, berries, red and green peppers, kiwi fruit, broccoli, baked potatoes, fortified juices.

Fat-soluble vitamins

The body absorbs fat-soluble vitamins through the intestines with the help of fats (lipids). The body can store them and does not remove them quickly. People who follow a low-fat diet may not be able to absorb enough of these vitamins. If too many build up, problems can arise.

Vitamin        Effect of too little      Effect of too much Sources

Vitamin A (retinoidsTrusted Source) Night        blindness Pressure on the brain, nausea, dizziness, skin irritation, joint and bone pain, orange pigmented skin color Sweet potato, beef liver, spinach, and other dark leafy greens, carrots, winter squash

Vitamin DTrusted Source     Poor bone formation and weak bones    Anorexia, weight loss, changes in heart rhythm, damage to cardiovascular system and kidneys

Sunlight exposure plus dietary sources: cod liver oil, oily fish, dairy products, fortified juices

Vitamin ETrusted Source        Peripheral         neuropathy, retinopathy, reduced immune response        May        reduce the ability of blood to clot        Wheatgerm,      nuts,      seeds, sunflower and safflower oil, spinach

Vitamin KTrusted Source       Bleeding  and  hemorrhaging in severe casesNo adverse effects but it may interact with blood thinners and other drugs        Leafy,            green vegetables, soybeans, edamame, okra, natto

Multivitamins are available for purchase in stores or online, but people should speak to their doctor before taking any supplements, to check that they are suitable for them to use.

Antioxidants

Some nutrients also act as antioxidants. These may be vitamins, minerals, proteins, or other types of molecules. They help the body remove toxic substances known as free radicals, or reactive oxygen species. If too many of these substances remain in the body, cell damage and disease can result.

# DIETITIAN VS. NUTRITIONIST

A registered dietitian nutritionist (RD or RDN) studies food, nutrition, and dietetics. To become a registered dietitian, a person needs to attend an accredited university, follow an approved curriculum, complete a rigorous internship, pass a licensure exam, and complete 75 or more continuing education hours every 5 years. Dietitians work in private and public healthcare, education, corporate wellness, research, and the food industry. A nutritionist learns about nutrition through self-study or formal education, but they do not meet the requirements to use the titles RD or RDN. Nutritionists often work in the food industry and in food science and technology.

# A LIST OF 50 SUPER HEALTHY FOODS

Eating a wide variety of nutritious foods, including fruit, vegetables, nuts, seeds, and lean protein can help support your overall health..Many foods are both healthy and tasty. By filling your plate with fruits, vegetables, quality protein sources, and other whole foods, you'll have meals that are colorful, versatile, and good for you. Here are 50 healthy and delicious to include in your diet.

1–6: Fruits and berries

Fruits and berries are popular health foods. They are sweet, nutritious, and easy to incorporate into your diet because they require little to no preparation.

1. Apples

Apples contain fiber, vitamin C, and numerous antioxidants. They are very filling and make the perfect snack if you're hungry between meals.

## 2. Avocados

Avocados are different from most other fruits because they contain lots of healthy fat. They are not only creamy and tasty but also high in fiber, potassium, and vitamin C. Swap mayonnaise for avocado as a salad dressing, or spread it on toast for breakfast.

## 3. Bananas

Bananas are a good source of potassium. They're also high in vitamin B6 and fiber and are convenient and portable.

## 4. Blueberries

Blueberries are both delicious and high in antioxidants.

## 5. Oranges

Oranges are well known for their vitamin C content. What's more, they're high in fiber and antioxidants.

## 6. Strawberries

Strawberries are highly nutritious and low in both carbs and calories. They provide vitamin C, fiber, and manganese and make a delicious dessert.

Other healthy fruits:

Other healthy fruits and berries include cherries, grapes, grapefruit, kiwi, lemons, mangoes, melons, olives, peaches, pears, pineapples, plums, and raspberries.

## 7. Eggs

Eggs are highly nutritious. Once demonized for being high in cholesterol, expertsTrusted Source now see them as a useful source of protein that may have various benefits.

## 8–10: Meats

Lean, unprocessed meats can be included in a healthy diet.

## 8. Lean beef

Lean beef is an excellent source of protein if you consume it in moderation. It also provides highly bioavailable iron.

## 9. Chicken breasts

Chicken breast is low in fat and calories but high in protein. It's a great source of many nutrients.

## 10. Lamb and mutton

Sheep are usually grass-fed, and their meat tends to be high inTrusted Source omega-3 fatty acids compared with omega-6.

## 11–15: Nuts and seeds

Despite being high in unsaturated fat and calories, nuts and seeds may help lower the riskTrusted Source of cardiovascular disease, cancer, and other health issues. They are a satisfying snack could help those managing their weight. They also require almost no preparation, so they're easy to add to your routine. They can also add texture to salads and other dishes. However, they are not suitable for people with a nut allergy.

## 11. Almonds

Almonds are a popular nut that contain with vitamin E, antioxidants, magnesium, and fiber. A 2021 reviewTrusted

Source found that almonds may contribute to weight loss, support the gut microbiota, improve thinking, manage heart rate when a person is under stress, and prevent skin aging.

## 12. Chia seeds

Chia seeds are a nutrient-dense addition to the diet. A single ounce (28 grams) provides 11 grams of fiber and significant amounts of magnesium, manganese, calcium, and various other nutrients.

## 13. Coconuts

Coconuts provide fiber and fatty acids called medium-chain triglycerides (MCTs).

## 14. Macadamia nuts

Macadamia nuts are tasty and higher in monounsaturated fats and lower in omega-6 fatty acids than most other nuts.

## 15. Walnuts

Walnuts are highly nutritious and rich in fiber and various vitamins and minerals. Pair them with feta cheese to dress a salad.

## 16. Brazil nuts

Brazil nuts are nutrient-rich and have a smooth, buttery texture. The nutrients they contain support thyroid function, and they are a good source of the mineral selenium.

## 17–26: Vegetables

Calorie for calorie, vegetables are among the most concentrated sources of nutrients. Including a variety of vegetables in your diet will ensure you get a wide range of nutrients.

## 17. Asparagus

Asparagus is a popular vegetable that is low in both carbs and calories and rich in vitamin K.

## 18. Bell peppers

Bell peppers come in several colors, including red, yellow, and green. They're crunchy and sweet and are a great source of antioxidants and vitamin C.

## 19. Broccoli

Broccoli is a cruciferous vegetable that tastes great both raw and cooked. It's an excellent source of fiber and vitamins C and K and contains a decent amount of protein compared with other vegetables.

20. Carrots

Carrots are a popular root vegetable. They're sweet, crunchy, and loaded with nutrients such as fiber and vitamin K. They're also high in carotene antioxidants, which have numerous benefits. Put a few carrots stick in your lunch box or use them for eating guacamole and other dips.

21. Cauliflower

Cauliflower is a very versatile cruciferous vegetable. You can add it to curries, roast it with olive oil, or use it raw in salads or for dipping.

22. Cucumber

Cucumbers make a refreshing snack. They are low in both carbs and calories, consisting mostly of water. They also contain small amounts of vitamin K and other nutrients.

23. Garlic

Garlic is a healthy and tasty addition to salads and cooked savory dishes. It containsTrusted Source allicin, which has antioxidant and antimicrobial effects. Its nutrients may also reduce the risk of cancer and cardiovascular disease.

24. Kale

Kale is high in fiber, vitamins C and K, and other nutrients. It adds a satisfying crunch to salads and other dishes. You can also add it to stir fries or bake in the oven to make crunchy kale chips.

25. Onions

Onions have a strong flavor and feature in many recipes. They contain a number of bioactive compounds believed to have health benefits.

## What are the 20 most healthy foods?

Research from 2021 developed a scoring system of food based on 54 attributes covering these nine domains:

nutrient ratios, vitamins, minerals, food ingredients, additives, processing, specific lipids, fiber and protein, and phytochemicals. Based on the mean values of this scoring system, the healthiest food categories are:

legumes

vegetables

fruit

fish and seafood

sauce condiment

dairy

mixed dishes

beverages

grains

meat, poultry, eggs

fats and oils

savory snacks and sweet desserts

Of course, whether a particular food is healthier than another ultimately depends on the exact food and any specific ingredients it may contain. It's a good idea to consult a dietician to determine exactly what foods are best for you.

*What foods are healthy to eat every day?*

According to the Dietary Guidelines for Americans 2020-2025, each day you should aim to eat a variety of fruit, vegetables, dairy, grains, and foods containing protein (either plant-based or from lean meats or fish).

*What is the #1 healthiest food?*

No one food can provide all the nutrients you need to consume in one day, so eating a balanced diet is the best way to get what you need to stay healthy. In addition, the state of your overall health and any conditions you might have may limit what foods you can consume, even if they are very nutritious. Speak to your doctor to determine the best nutrition plan for you. That said, research looking at the nutrient density of various food groups found that the following foods contain the most nutrients:

organ meats

small fish

dark green leafy vegetables

bivalves such as oysters and clams

crustaceans such as lobster and shrimp

goat meat

beef

eggs

milk

canned fish with bones

mutton

lamb

The bottom line

Whether you want to overhaul your diet or simply change up your meals, it's easy to add a number of these foods to your routine. Many of the foods above make a great snack while also providing essential nutrients. Some may even aid weight loss.

# 14 'HEALTH FOODS' THAT MAY NOT BE AS NUTRITIOUS AS YOU THOUGHT

Navigating the grocery aisles in search of nutritious foods has become increasingly complex as an increasingly large number of so-called healthy products fill the shelves. Companies often use wording on product labels and in their marketing to appeal to customers who are trying to make healthier choices. You might see claims on labels like:

- low fat

- vegan

- gluten-free

- low carb

Unfortunately, just because a food uses words like these on its label or is generally thought of as healthier than other foods doesn't mean it's good for you. Here are 14 foods that may not be as healthy as their marketing claims make them out to be.

1. Granola and granola bars

People have championed granola and granola bars as "healthy" foods for decades. Even though some granolas and granola bars are quite nutritious, many are packed with added sugar and very high in calories. For example, a 2/3-cup (67-gram) serving of Nature Valley Oats and Dark Chocolate Protein Granola contains 7 grams of added sugar and 290 calories, while Quaker Chewy Yogurt Granola Bars pack 10 grams of added sugar per bar  The recommended Daily Value (DV) for sugar is 50 grams for a person who consumes 2,000 calories per day, according to the Food and Drug Administration. For optimal health, it's best to limit your added sugar intake as much as possible, as consuming too much added sugar can contribute to an increased risk of many health conditions in both adults and kids. These health conditions include:

obesity

fatty liver

heart disease

Instead of buying premade granola at the store, try making your own granola and granola bars at home. You can use nutritious ingredients like nuts and oats and add sweetness with dried fruit.

2. Flavored yogurts

Yogurt can be a healthy choice, but it's best to opt for unsweetened yogurt whenever possible. Flavored and "fruit on the bottom" yogurts can contain a surprising amount of sugar in just a small serving. For example, a 5.3-ounce (150-gram) container of Dannon Strawberry Fruit on the Bottom yogurt contains a hefty 15 grams of added sugar. Yogurts that have candy toppings and "flip-style" yogurts can have even more. Instead of choosing sweetened yogurt, try topping unsweetened yogurt with fresh fruit for a bit of natural sweetness.

3. Protein drinks and bars

Many people are under the impression that the higher the protein content of a food or beverage, the healthier it is. Some foods that are naturally high in protein, like fish, eggs, and beans, are without a doubt healthy choices. However, items like protein bars and protein shakes may not be as healthy as some people assume. Many healthy people who consume balanced diets don't need to get extra protein through supplements. Nevertheless, active individuals and those who follow vegetarian and vegan diets may benefit from more protein in their diets.

If you do need extra protein, you may be able to get this by eating more protein-rich foods. As such, for many people, eating supplemental protein products like bars and drinks may not be necessary to stay healthy (9Trusted Source). Plus, many of these items are loaded with added sugar and unnecessary ingredients, like:

artificial sweeteners

artificial colors

oils

thickeners

4. Sports drinks and energy beverages

While companies market sports drinks and energy beverages as ways to boost energy and athletic performance, these beverages are unnecessary for most people. They can also be high in ingredients like added sugar, artificial colors, and large amounts of stimulants, such as caffeine..While some athletes do need to replenish lost nutrients with sports drinks after intense exercise, most people who perform moderate exercise or just normal daily activity do not need to chug sports drinks to stay hydrated. Many sports beverages contain a shocking amount of sugar. For example, a 20-ounce (591-mL) bottle of Fruit Punch Gatorade contains 34 grams of added sugar. Likewise, energy drinks can be extremely high in added sugar. The popular Monster Energy drink contains 54 grams per 16-ounce (473-mL) can. That's higher than the DV for added sugar .

These beverages are heavily marketed toward children and adolescents, which is alarming because researchers have linked drinking sweetened beverages with health issues, including high blood pressure, fatty liver, and obesity, in kids and teens.

5. Gluten-free snack foods

For people with gluten-related disorders, avoiding gluten is necessary. However, even if a food is labeled as gluten-free, it's not necessarily healthier than gluten-containing foods. Some processed gluten-free snack foods and sweets contain just as much, if not more, calories and added sugar as other snacks. Additionally, studies show that gluten-free snack foods and other gluten-free items tend to be lower in protein, fiber, and certain vitamins and minerals than their gluten-containing counterparts. They're also generally more expensive.

6. Some low fat and fat-free products

Just because a food is low in fat doesn't mean it's a healthier choice. Food manufacturers often replace fat with sugar in low fat and fat-free products to make up for the flavor loss. What's more, fat-free products may be less filling than their full fat versions because fat is a macronutrient that supports feelings of fullness and makes food more pleasurable to eat. Fats are an essential part of your diet and eating nutritious high fat foods can help you reap their benefits.

7. Breakfast cereal

Many people assume that breakfast cereals are a smart way to start their day. However, this isn't always the case. In fact, many breakfast cereals are made with refined grains, lack filling nutrients like protein and fiber, and can be very high in added sugar. Even cereals marketed toward adults can be packed with added sugar. Honey Nut Cheerios, which is marketed as "heart healthy," contains 12 grams of added sugar per cup. Eating large amounts of cereal like this one, particularly as part of a diet that's already high in added sugar, doesn't promote heart health. In fact, diets high in added sugar likely have the opposite effect. Studies have linked high sugar diets to an increased risk of heart disease and heart disease risk factors, including high blood pressure and triglyceride levels.

8. Some vegetable oils

Your body needs both omega-6 fats and omega-3 fats — like eicosapentaenoic acid (EPA) and docosahexaenoic acid (DHA) — to function. Unfortunately, modern-day diets have a ratio of about 20:1, far exceeding the body's needs for omega-6 fats. Research has found that this imbalance in the omega-6 to omega-3 ratio is associated with systemic inflammation, and studies suggest it may contribute to disease risk.

Most people who eat a Western diet consume too much omega-6-rich fat and not enough omega-3s. For this reason, it's best to limit your intake of foods high in omega-6 fats. These include:

soybean oil

corn oil

sunflower oil

products made with these oils, including many processed, prepackaged foods

Another solution is to increase your intake of omega-3s. Good sources of omega-3s include:

flaxseed oil

fatty fish, like salmon

walnuts

9. Premade smoothies

efetova/Getty Images

Homemade smoothies can be a nutritious choice and convenient way to increase your consumption of fruits and vegetables. Yet, premade smoothies and smoothies from certain chain restaurants contain massive amounts of calories and sugar. If you buy a smoothie when you're out and about, make sure to read the ingredient label before you order. Many smoothie stores offer items made with frozen yogurt, sherbet, and other sugar-laden additives.

## 10. Diet soda

Even though diet soda contains no sugar and generally zero calories, studies show that those who drink diet soda regularly are more likely to develop certain health issues than people who don't drink it. For example, it's also associated with a higher risk of metabolic syndrome, a group of symptoms that include increased belly fat, blood sugar, blood pressure, and blood fat levels. Research suggests that diet soda may contribute to these health issues by altering brain responses to food, increasing the desire for highly palatable foods like calorie-dense sweets.

## 11. Some plant-based meat products

Following a plant-centric diet and eating less meat can benefit your overall health, as well as the environment. However, some vegan and plant-based meat replacement products are packed with ultra-processed ingredients, salt, sugar, and more. Instead of relying on store-bought vegan meat products, try using whole-food ingredients to make your own at home. For example, you can make plant-based burgers out of ingredients like black beans, mushrooms, rice, and cashews.

12. Frozen yogurt

While frozen yogurt (also known as fro-yo) may be delicious, it's not always a healthier choice than regular ice cream. Frozen yogurt is generally lower in fat than ice cream, but it can be very high in added sugar. Plus, most self-serve fro-yo establishments only provide large cups, which customers tend to fill. These stores also offer a variety of high calorie, sugary toppings, which can add significant amounts of added sugar and drive up the calorie count of your dessert. While it's perfectly acceptable to enjoy ice cream or frozen yogurt on occasion, one isn't necessarily a healthier choice than the other. Choose whichever you prefer and consider sticking to smaller portion sizes to keep your calorie and added sugar intake in check.

## 13. Yogurt-covered pretzels and raisins

Yogurt-covered snacks like pretzels and raisins are sold in most health food stores and sometimes marketed as a healthier choice than chocolate-covered snacks. However, they're very similar nutritionally. A 100-gram serving of yogurt-covered raisins contains 393 calories and 64 grams of total sugar, while the same serving of raisins covered in milk chocolate contains 390 calories and 62.2 grams of total sugar. Still, note that the sugar and calorie contents vary by brand.

## 14. Some plant-based milks

Plant milks have grown in popularity as more people transition to a more plant-based diet. Even though nut milk can be an excellent alternative to dairy products, especially for those who are intolerant to milk products, some nut milks may not be as healthy as you think. Unless explicitly stated on the bottle, most plant milks contain added sugar to improve their taste. For example, original Almond

Breeze almond milk contains 7 grams of added sugar per 1-cup (240-mL) serving, with cane sugar listed as the second ingredient. For this reason, it's a good idea to choose unsweetened nut milks if you want to moderate your intake of added sugar. Even though food companies market many foods and beverages as "healthy," some may not be nutritious choices. Many of these foods are packed with added sugar and other ingredients that may negatively affect your overall health. Plus, many foods marketed as "healthier" options are much more expensive than other products.

This is why it's important to always read the label to investigate the nutrition facts and ingredients of food products, including those marketed as "healthy." And, in general, try to stick mostly to whole, nutrient-dense foods. Just one thing;

*Try this today:*
Revise your approach to grocery shopping. If you're interested in improving your diet quality, there's no need to purchase "health foods." Instead, focus on adding more foods to your diet that are strongly linked to improved diet quality and health outcomes. Whole foods are your best bet,

including vegetables, fruits, nuts, seeds, spices, beans, and fish.

Grocery stores most often stock whole foods around the perimeter of the store, so sticking mostly to the perimeter is one good trick when you're at the supermarket.

Meanwhile, reduce your intake of ultra-processed foods, such as fast food, soda, and candy. These and so-called health foods are often located in the center aisles of the grocery store.

## 9 High-Fat Foods That Offer Great Health Benefits

Certain high fat foods, including dairy products, eggs, and plants like avocados, pack important nutrients that can benefit your health. Many contain protein, fiber, and key vitamins. Although dietary fat was once avoided and considered a major contributor to heart disease, researchers have found that it can offer some benefits. However, the American Heart AssociationTrusted Source recommends that saturated fat should be limited to less than 10% of total calorie intake. Though some saturated fats — like those found in dairy — may not have the same negative effect as saturated fats that are found in red meat. Still, full-fat foods may offer benefits over their reduced-fat or fat-free counterparts. They are usually less processed and lower in sugar and carbs. Here are 9 high-fat foods that are incredibly nutritious;

Avocados

AvocadosTrusted Source are unique in the world of fruits. Whereas most fruits primarily contain carbs, avocados are loaded with fats. In fact, avocados are about 80% fat, by calories, making them even higher in fat than most animal foods. Avocados are also among the best sources of potassium in the diet, providing 15% of the Daily Value (DV) per 5-ounce (150-gram) serving. In addition, they're packed with antioxidant compounds.

Additionally, one study involving 45 men and women found that consuming one avocado daily for 5 weeks had favorable effects on participants' cholesterol profiles.

They're also a great source of fiber, which offers numerous digestive, heart health, and weight management benefits.

Cheese

Cheese is surprisingly nutritious, despite its iffy reputation. It is a great source of calcium, vitamin B12, phosphorus, and selenium and contains many other nutrients. It is also rich in protein, with a single ounce (28 grams) of cheese containing 6 grams of protein, nearly as much as a glass of milk. Cheese, like other high-fat dairy products, also doesn't appear to increase heart disease risk compared with reduced-fat dairy — as it was previously thought to.

Dark chocolate

Dark chocolateTrusted Source is a nutritious food disguised as a tasty treat. It is very high in fat, with fat accounting for around 65% of calories. It's important to choose dark chocolate with at least 70% cocoa, as other varieties are higher in added sugar and lower in the nutrients and antioxidants that dark chocolate provides. In addition, dark chocolate contains fiber and several notable nutrients, including iron and magnesium, which some people may have difficulty getting enough of. It is also loaded with antioxidants like resveratro, the same antioxidant that gives red wine its health benefits, and epicatechin, which may possess anti-aging and performance-enhancing properties.

Whole eggs

Whole eggs used to be considered unhealthy because the yolks are high in cholesterol and fat. However, new studiesTrusted Source have shown that cholesterol in eggs does not negatively affect the cholesterol in the blood, at least not in the majority of people. In addition, eggs are nutrient-dense, containing a variety of vitamins and minerals. One example is cholineTrusted Source, a nutrient that is essential for brain and nerve health. One egg (50 gramsTrusted Source) provides 27% of the DV of choline. Eggs are also a weight-loss–friendly food. They are high in protein, which can help you to stay fuller between meals and cut down on excess calories. Yolks and all, eggs can be a healthy addition to any diet.

Fatty fish

Fatty fish is widely regarded as one of the most nutritious animal protein sources available. This includes fish like salmonTrusted Source, trout, anchovies, mackerel, sardines, and herring. These fish are loaded with heart-healthy omega-3 fatty acids, high quality proteins, and a variety of vitamins and minerals. Research shows that regular fatty fish consumption may enhance cognitive functionTrusted Source, help regulate blood sugar levelsTrusted Source, and decrease heart disease risk. If you can't (or don't) eat fish, taking a fish oil supplement may be useful. Cod fish liver oil is best. It contains all the omega-3s that you need, as well as plenty of vitamin D.


Nuts

NutsTrusted Source are incredibly healthy. They are high in healthy fats and fiber and are a good plant-based source of protein. Nuts also contain vitamin E and are loaded with magnesium, a mineral that most people don't get enough of.

Studies show  that people who eat nuts tend to have a lower rate of obesity and a lower risk of heart disease. Healthy nuts include almonds, walnuts, macadamia nuts, and numerous others.

Chia seeds

Chia seeds  are generally not thought of as a "fatty" food, but an ounce (28 grams) of chia seeds actually contains 11 grams of fat. Additionally, almost all the carbs in chia seeds are fiber — so the vast majority of calories in them actually come from fat. These aren't just any fats either. The majority of the fats in chia seeds consist of the heart-healthy, essential omega-3 fatty acid called alpha-linolenic acid (ALA). Chia seeds may also have numerous health benefits, such as lowering blood pressure and having anti-inflammatory effects. They are also incredibly nutritious. In addition to being loaded with fiber and omega-3s, chia seeds are also packed with nutrients.

Extra virgin olive oil

Another fatty food that almost everyone agrees is healthy is extra virgin olive oil. It's high in oleic acid , a fatty acid with powerful anti-inflammatory properties. This fat is an essential component of the Mediterranean diet, which has been shown to have numerous health benefits regarding heart health, blood sugar management, and weight management. It's extremely versatile in cooking but really shines on roasted vegetables and in homemade salad dressings.


Full-fat yogurt

Full-fat yogurt can be nutrient rich. It has all the same important nutrients as other high-fat dairy products. However, it's also loaded with healthy probiotics that can have powerful effects on your health. Studies show that yogurt may improve digestive healthTrusted Source and may even help with weight managementTrusted Source and reducing heart disease riskTrusted Source. Additionally, research suggests that full-fat dairy has no negative health effects compared with fat-free or reduced-fat dairy. It's important to choose full-fat or whole-milk yogurt and select a version with minimal added sugar. Although high-fat foods were once thought to be low in nutrients, research now shows that some fats do not pose the negative concerns for heart health that it once thought to. Additionally, naturally, high-fat foods may offer similar health benefits to their low fat counterparts while being less processed. Although they are higher in calories, the high fat foods on this list can easily be part of a nutrient-dense, whole–food–based diet.

# CULTURAL COMPETENCE IN NUTRITION AND DIETETICS: WHAT WE NEED TO KNOW

Culture refers to the ideas, customs, and behaviors of a group of people or a society. It influences just about everything you do — the way you speak, the foods you eat, what you consider to be right or wrong, your religious and spiritual practices, and even your perspective of wellness, healing, and healthcare. However, culture is a complex and fluid concept with numerous ethnocultural communities, identities, and cross-cultural practices (1, 3). This diversity presents a challenge to the healthcare industry and providers, who must be adequately trained and skilled to include the nuances of culture in their consultations and recommendations.

In the field of dietetics, culturally appropriate nutrition guidelines and nutrition therapy recommendations are essential. The absence of cultural competence among dietitians may perpetuate health inequities and disparities among marginalized and diverse communities.

## What is cultural competence?

Cultural competence is the willingness and ability to treat a patient effectively and appropriately without the influence of bias, prejudice, or stereotypes. It requires respecting others' attitudes, beliefs, and values while evaluating your own and becoming comfortable with any differences that arise. Differences are often seen in race, ethnicity, religion, and food practices. As a framework developed in the 1980s, cultural competence in the health industry seeks to make healthcare services more acceptable, accessible, relatable, and effective for individuals from diverse backgrounds.

In nutrition, it's a group of strategies meant to address cultural diversity and challenge the cookie-cutter approach to nutrition education and dietary interventions among ethnocultural communities. This includes nutrition guidelines and illustrations representing diverse food cultures with an expanded definition of "healthy eating." It involves nutritionists and dietitians knowledgeable and skilled in cultural counseling techniques including culture in the discussions and recommendations. They provide unbiased nutrition services that do not undermine culture's influence on lifestyle, food choices, and eating patterns. Cultural competence overlaps with cultural sensitivity, awareness, and cultural safety, encompassing more than just race/ethnicity and religion, and it's careful not to mislabel based on stereotypes. A major aim of cultural competence is to build a system of trained healthcare professionals capable of providing tailored, culturally appropriate expertise. Cultural competence is a framework developed to make healthcare services more accessible and effective for diverse ethnic communities. It's a group of strategies that challenge the approach to nutrition education and dietary interventions.

## Why is cultural competence in dietetics important?

Social determinants of health must be interpreted and understood within the context of systemic racism and how it affects different cultures and ethnicities  These determinants — including socioeconomic status, education,

food insecurity, housing, employment, and food access —
lead to social gradients and health inequities. These health
inequities and subsequent health disparities are amplified
among marginalized, red-lined, and underserved
populations who may lack access to nutritious foods and
food security. Culture also influences the client's
perspective on health and healing, their use of medication
versus alternative therapies, and their food choices and
eating patterns. Models of cultural competence exist and
are promoted through nutrition textbooks, practicums, and
internships to improve dietitians' skills related to
addressing ethnocultural diversity.

However, clinical practice guidelines, meal planning,
healthy eating, and medical nutrition therapy are often
presented in a decontextualized manner. The encounter
between dietitian and patient is shaped by the differences in
their cultures, biases, prejudices, and stereotypes. If a
dietitian does not effectively manage these differences, a
breakdown in trust, communication, and compliance with
the nutrition plan may further propagate poor health
outcomes.

Dietitians and nutritionists must acknowledge these diverse influences to cultivate an atmosphere of trust and develop an affinity with patients, enabling them to communicate an effective nutrition plan and yield greater compliance and good health outcomes. Furthermore, healthy eating looks different across ethnocultural communities and geographical locations based on food accessibility, sustainability, and food cultures. Health disparities may develop if dietitians fail to give culturally competent nutrition interventions.

And while cultural competency is not a panacea for health disparities, more thorough communication with the client promotes better health outcome. Nutrition advice needs to be responsive, appropriate, and effectively matched to the client's lifestyle, living conditions, dietary needs, and food culture. As such, cultural competence is a crucial skill for dietitians and healthcare professionals alike. To address health inequities and disparities, the social determinants of health must be understood within the context of culture and reflected through unbiased, culturally appropriate, and respectful nutrition services.

## What happens in the absence of cultural competence?

Below are some real-life scenarios that observe the breakdown in communication that cultural barriers can cause due to inadequate or inappropriate cultural competence. While reviewing these scenarios, you can consider solutions that could improve the outcome of similar future events.

At the individual level

Performing a self-assessment of your own beliefs, values, biases, prejudices, and stereotypes is the first step to becoming culturally competent. Be cognizant of what you bring to the table — both positive and negative biases — and become comfortable with the differences that may arise between you and someone from a different ethnocultural background.

People do not need to be the same to be respected. Here's a list to help you get started:

Address your personal biases and prejudices by reflecting on your own belief system.

Acknowledge the differences that your clients may have, but do not pass judgment, remaining neutral instead.

Ask permission instead of lecturing the patient. Asking, "Do you mind if we spoke about [insert cultural topic/behavior]" communicates respect for the patient, and they are more likely to be engaged.

Develop culturally appropriate interventions that are specific to the patient and not a stereotype of their ethnicity.

At the institutional level

The forms of help that are available in a healthcare system reflect the value it places on cultural knowledge and practices. The inability to access culturally appropriate nutrition and dietary services is a form of social inequity and health disparity. Institutions can seek to improve how they engage with and empower members of marginalized communities. Here are some suggestions for improving cultural competence at the institutional level:

Hire a diverse staff that's representative of the ethnocultural diversity of the patient population.

Ethnic matching of dietitian and patient may help the patient feel safe and understood.

Create standards of practice that encourage dietitians to develop culturally adapted interventions or offer patients interventions drawn from their own cultural tradition as part of the care plan.

Possibly refer to other sources of healing that are safe and align with the patient's cultural practices.

Include nutrition guidelines that consider food cultures, including one-pot meals, as these are a part of several immigrant and ethnocultural dietary patterns.

Change is required at both individual and institutional levels to build culturally competent nutritionists and dietitians and a supportive healthcare environment capable of reducing health disparities.

*Does cultural competence go far enough?*

Some literature suggests that cultural competence is insufficient — that simply making nutritionists and dietitians aware of cultural differences is not enough to stop stereotyping and affect change. Furthermore, some cultural competence movements may be purely cosmetic or superficial. The concepts of cultural safety and cultural humility have been proposed as more inclusive and systematic approaches to dismantling institutional discrimination (1). Cultural safety looks beyond an individual dietitian's skills to create a work environment that's a safe cultural space for the patient, one that's sensitive and responsive to their various belief systems. Meanwhile, cultural humility is viewed as a more reflexive approach, going beyond just acquiring knowledge and involves an ongoing self-exploration and self-critique process, combined with a willingness to learn from others.

To demean or disempower a patient's cultural identity is considered a culturally unsafe practice. However, although some patients may feel safe and understood concerning institutional cultural competence and ethnic matching of dietitian and patient, others may feel singled out and exposed to racial prejudice. Implementation of cultural competence in clinical practice may also extend consultation times, as it requires more dialogue with the patient. Interestingly, not every non-Western practice is going to be the best intervention. It's essential to move away from the notion that any one style of eating is bad — the way Western eating has been demonized — to addressing eating patterns that may be harmful regardless of origin. There are downsides to cultural competence that create further challenges to institutionalizing it, including cosmetic movements, lack of inclusivity, and unintentional prejudice.

## Organizations advocating for cultural competence in dietetics

Within the Academy of Nutrition and Dietetics (AND) and independent organizations, several Member Interest Groups advocate diversifying nutrition to make it inclusive. These include:

The National Organization of Blacks in Dietetics (NOBIDAN). This professional association provides a forum for the professional development and support of dietetics, optimal nutrition, and well-being for the general public, especially those of African descent.

Latinos and Hispanics in Dietetics and Nutrition (LAHIDAN). Their mission is to empower members to be food and nutrition leaders for Latinos and Hispanics.

The Asian American and Pacific Islanders (AAPI) and Indians in Nutrition and Dietetics (IND). Their main values are advocating for cultural topics and cultural approaches in nutrition and dietetics.

Diversify Dietetics (DD). They aim to increase racial and ethnic diversity in nutrition by empowering nutrition leaders of color and assisting aspiring dietitians of color with financial aid and internship applications.

Dietitians for food justice. This Canadian network of dietitians, dietetic interns, and students addresses food injustices. Members work to create an anti-racist and health equity approach to food access in Toronto and beyond.

Growing Resilience in the South (GRITS). A nonprofit bridging the gap between nutrition and culture by providing free nutrition counseling to vulnerable populations and programs for dietitians and students to improve their understanding of African American cultural foods.

Member Interest Groups and other non-academy organizations are pivoting dietitians' roles as advocates of cultural competence in dietetics and food access.

Cultural competence is the willingness and ability to provide unbiased, judgment-free nutrition services to people and clients of diverse cultural backgrounds. Cultural competence and cultural safety intersect and demand institutional changes to facilitate the forms of help available to minority and marginalized communities. However, culture is a fluid concept, and nutritionists and dietitians must not assume that every member of a specific ethnic group identifies and complies with that group's commonly known cultural practices. They may have adapted their own values and practices. Dietitians should remain impartial and engage clients in meaningful conversations that will equip them with the information they need to provide culturally appropriate, respectful guidance.

## Healthy Eating Includes Cultural Foods

On one hand, it's essential to good health, but on the other, it's suggestive of restriction and self-denial steeped in Eurocentrism. Even in the Caribbean, where I'm from, many nutrition programs are modeled on the American food pyramid, which then implies what healthy eating looks like to the local communities. However, nutrition and healthy eating are not a one-size-fits-all dietary prescription. Traditional meals and food culture deserve a seat at the table too.

*What are cultural foods?*

Cultural foods — also called traditional dishes — represent the traditions, beliefs, and practices of a geographic region, ethnic group, religious body, or cross-cultural community. Cultural foods may involve beliefs about how certain foods are prepared or used. They may also symbolize a group's overall culture. These dishes and customs are passed down from generation to generation.

Cultural foods may represent a region, such as pizza, pasta, and tomato sauce from Italy or kimchi, seaweed, and dim sum from Asia. Alternatively, they may represent a colonial past, such as the fusion of West African and East Indian food traditions throughout the Caribbean. Cultural foods may play a part in religious celebrations and are often at the core of our identities and familial connections.

Cultural foods must be fully integrated into the Western framework

Healthy eating includes cultural foods — but that message isn't prominent and often goes unapplied..The U.S. Department of Agriculture's (USDA) Dietary Guidelines for Americans is one of the gold standards for nutrition guidelines in the West. It recommends meeting people where they are — including their cultural foodways. The Canadian Food Guide also emphasizes the importance of culture and food traditions to healthy eating. However, the field of dietetics still has a lot of work to do to ensure cultural competence, which is the effective and appropriate treatment of people without bias, prejudice, or stereotypes. During my training to become a dietitian, cultural needs and food practices were acknowledged, but there was limited interest or practical application. In some instances, there were few institutional resources for healthcare professionals.

## What does healthy eating really look like?

Healthy eating is loosely defined as the consumption of a variety of nutrients from dairy, protein foods, grains, fruits, and vegetables — what's known in the United States as the five food groups. The main message is that each food group provides essential vitamins and minerals needed to support good health. The USDA's MyPlate, which replaced the food pyramid, illustrates that a healthy plate is half nonstarchy vegetables, one-quarter protein, and one-quarter grains. However, the Caribbean is a melting pot of six food groups — staples (starchy, carb-rich foods), foods from animals, legumes, fruits, vegetables, and fats or oils (5).

Traditional one-pot dishes can't always be distinctly portioned on a plate. Rather, the food groups are combined into a single dish. For example, the traditional one-pot dish called oil down is made with breadfruit (the staple — a starchy fruit that has a texture similar to bread once cooked), nonstarchy veggies like spinach and carrots, and meats like chicken, fish, or pork.

Dietary guidelines demonstrate that cultural foods go hand in hand with healthy eating. However, improved cultural competence and institutional resources are needed to facilitate the practical application of these guidelines.

Healthy eating is much more fluid than what you see online

Your desire to eat certain foods is often the result of targeted and successful food marketing. This marketing usually comes through a Eurocentric lens that lacks cultural nuance. For instance, Googling "healthy eating" reveals a flurry of lists and images of asparagus, blueberries, and Atlantic salmon — often in the arms or on the tables of a white family. The lack of cultural representation or ethnically diverse illustrations sends an unspoken message that local and cultural foods may be unhealthy. Yet, true healthy eating is a fluid concept that neither has a specific look or ethnicity nor needs to include specific foods to count. Here are foods you'll commonly see on health websites in the West, plus some traditional-food counterparts:

While kale is a nutritious vegetable, so too are dasheen bush (taro leaves) and spinach.

Quinoa is an excellent source of protein and dietary fiber, but rice and beans are too.

Chicken breast is low in fat and lauded as a must-have for a healthy diet, but if you remove the skin from other parts of the chicken, those pieces are low in fat too — and higher in iron.

Atlantic salmon is rich in omega-3 fatty acids, but so too are local salmon varieties and other fatty fish such as sardines.

If kale, quinoa, and Atlantic salmon aren't available in your region, your diet isn't automatically poor. Contrary to mainstream health and wellness messages, a healthy plate isn't limited to Eurocentric foods, and traditional foods aren't inferior or nutritionally unfit.

Healthy eating looks different across communities and locations based on food access, sustainability, and food cultures. Healthy eating is a fluid concept that looks different based on your region and cultural background. Its messaging needs to be diversified.

# CONCLUSION

Nutrition is the study of food and how it affects the body. People need to consume a varied diet to obtain a wide range of nutrients. Some people choose to follow a specific diet, in which they focus on certain foods and avoid others. People who do this may need to plan carefully to ensure they obtain all the necessary vitamins to maintain their health. A diet that is rich in plant-based foods and that limits added animal fats, processed foods, and added sugar and salt is most likely to benefit a person's health.